Acid Reflux:

What it is, causes, and natural health advice with recipes included

Eve Bell

Table of Contents

Disclaimer

While all attempts have been made to verify the information provided in this book, the author does assume any responsibility for errors, omissions, or contrary interpretations of the subject matter contained within. The information provided in this book is for educational and entertainment purposes only. The reader is responsible for his or her own actions and the author does not accept any responsibilities for any liabilities or damages, real or perceived, resulting from the use of this information.

The trademarks that are used are without any consent, and the publication of the trademark is without permission or backing by the trademark owner. All trademarks and brands within this book are for clarifying purposes only and are the owned by the owners themselves, not affiliated with this document.

You've tried everything...

Repeated doctor's visits, mints, online advice, and even avoiding foods just seem to be either temporary or don't work at all. You're tired of trying to regulate your reflux with prescription medications and then having to cope with the side effects. The problem is your reflux keeps coming back. You've looked online for help, but have either gotten bad advice or mixed information. If you're ready to get a handle on your reflux, then this book will walk you through everything from what it truly is to natural health advice and recipes you can make at home to finally get a handle on your condition.

Your feet are on the path...

If you are ready to get control of your reflux, then you've purchased the right book. This book was authored to answer the questions other resources could not or didn't answer them well enough to satisfy your curiosity. This book will take a deeper look into:

- What reflux is
- Why prescription medications can it worse
- Which foods are best left alone
- Which herbs can help with reflux.
- How to combine herbs into recipes for more effectiveness

Chapter 1 - What is Acid Reflux?

Most people would assume it's the burning sensation you get in your chest that can be anywhere from a mild annoyance to a debilitating pain so intense all you can do is squeeze yourself tightly and moan. When in fact, that's only part of it.

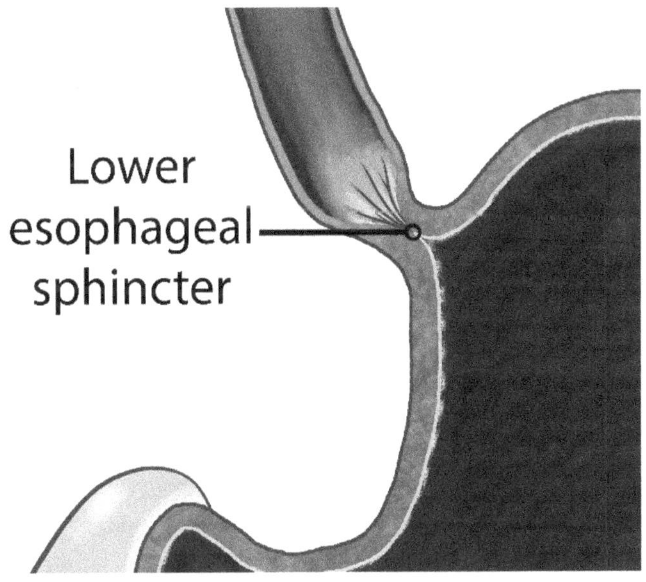

There is an opening at the top of the stomach called the esophageal sphincter. This is the part of the stomach which opens to allow entering the stomach but preventing the digestive acids from entering the esophagus. However, when you suffer from reflux, the LES does not shut completely, allowing some of the acids to backup into the esophagus.

This is commonly known as Acid Reflux Disease, but it is also classified as Gastroesophageal Reflux Disease. Most people who suffer from acid reflux also suffer from hiatal hernia. A hiatal hernia is when the upper stomach and LES shift above the diaphragm. One of the symptoms of hiatal hernia is the feeling of something getting "stuck" in your throat.

Now that we know what it is, we need to get to the root causes of how it comes to be and what can trigger it.

• Not eating for a long period of time. This is not a common cause, but it does happen. The best way to prevent reflux due to this is to eat small meals and snacks through the day.

• Stress is a factor. When you are in a high stress situation or in a situation that prolongs stress, it tends to wear down the weakest system in the body. If you have always had a weak digestive system, then it can turn into either an intestinal illness or acid reflux.

• Eating large portion meals can cause reflux. It's better to make portion sizes which are nutritionally balanced. At first glance, the portions will look small, but then you put it all together for a meal, it can be a lot of food.

• Lying down immediately after eating can also contribute to reflux. It generally takes a minimum of three hours to digest most of the food you eat at mealtime. Lying down can slow the digestive process, and if your LES does not close completely, the acid can leak into the esophagus.

• Obesity or being overweight can contribute to reflux. Being overweight puts pressure on the body, and the more fat you have on your body, the more it compresses your internal organs, making them work harder. It works the same with your stomach.

• Eating rich foods in meal and then lying down, even bending over can make the acid leak into the esophagus. Eating rich foods, like pasts dishes or other heavy foods can make you feel tired. This is due to your body rerouting the energy to help with digestion. Eat smaller portions of the rich foods to avoid the food coma and you should be okay.

• Eating is to close to bedtime. This one is related to lying down shortly after eating. It is always recommended that the last meal of the day should be eaten no later than six in the evening. This will give your digestive system time to work its magic.

• Eating foods high in citric acid, tomatoes, garlic, onions, even spicy and fatty foods can trigger it. Some can't eat minty foods. Your food triggers may vary from someone else. In order to find your triggers, make a journal of the foods you eat that give you reflux. In the case of orange juice, try the juice fresh, not from concentrate to see if that helps prevent a flare-up. The same goes for drinks like alcohol and so forth.

• Being a smoker can cause flare-ups as well.

• If you are pregnant, there is a chance you may have instances of reflux.

• Certain medications can cause it, too (especially, non-steroidal anti-inflammatory drugs or antibiotics).

- You may also have food allergy and don't know about it. Reflux can be a manifestation of food allergy, then it would be better to make an analysis IgG4 testing food intolerance and then exclude allergens (by the way it can help you not only fight a reflux, but improve your health. maybe you don't know about your individual intolerance to some healthy products because sometimes it doesn't have immediate reactions)

- Peptic ulcer disease and Gastritis (both of them can be caused by some factors such as Helicobacter Pylori or Inherited factors)
These are the most common reasons.

There is some advice on how to help yourself, but don't forget if you want to fight a disease you must find a reason. **So it's better to start from a medical examination.**

A note on prescriptions for reflux

If you are prescribed medications for acid reflux, you may find that running out will make the condition worse. This is due to the medicine's design of shutting off some of the valves that produce the acid. When the medication leaves your system, the valves will re-activate, causing a worse episode than before you started taking it. Your body is overcompensating. I am not telling you stop taking the medication, just advising you that this may be a cause of how it seems to be worse when you run out.

Serious Signs

Regular reflux can be managed by diet and some medications, but there are instances where you may need to take more drastic steps to keep your reflux regulated. Here are some symptoms to look out for:

• Constant bloating no matter what you eat. To give your doctor a better idea of the severity, mark down when you experience bloating.

• If your stools are bloody and/or black or if you have blood in your vomit. See a physician immediately.

• Constant burping. This may be related to bloating.

• Unrelenting hiccups.

• When your esophagus narrows and gives you a feeling of food being stuck.

• If you start losing weight for no reason, you need to contact your physician.

• If you have a constant sore throat, you wheeze, have a dry cough or are constantly hoarse.

• Being constantly nauseated.

Chapter 2 - The Digestive System

We are going to go a little deeper into how the gastrointestinal tract and how to maintain a balance to prevent reflux and other digestive problems.

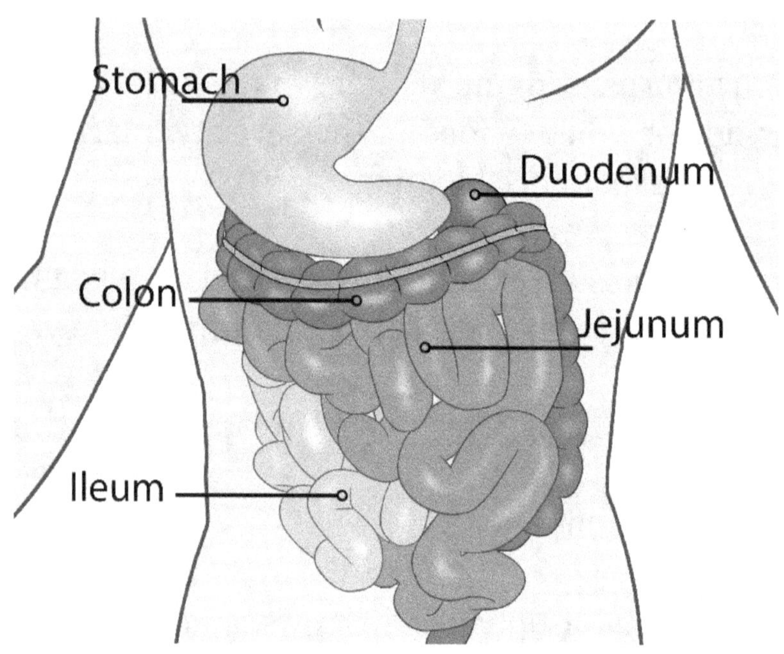

The Stomach

This is the first stop any food and drink taken in makes before continuing its journey. It is met with stomach acids and enzymes to break down the food and drink:

Pepsin, renni, hydrochloric acid, and mucus are the main acids and enzymes which make digestion happen in the stomach. Pepsin converts protein to make the substance easily absorbed. The hydrochloric acid helps the pepsin do the conversion. The rennin helps the stomach breakdown milk proteins. Mucus coats the lining of the stomach to protect the lining from the gastric juices. Hormones and certain chemical substances tend to stimulate acid and enzyme secretion. Only 10 percent of the digestive process is in the stomach.

The Small Intestine and Duodenum

As the substances in stomach get digested, they make their way to the small intestine. The rest of the digestion happens here, in the small intestine. It is here where the absorption of food and nutrients occurs. This is where the bulk of the enzymes and bile acids break down the foods to get them ready for adsorption. Once absorbed, the nutrients are conveyed to the blood stream and other parts of the body.

Colon

This is also known as the large intestine. The rest of the food is pushed here to travel to the anus.

PH Balance of the Digestive System

As scientists test certain substances for pH, your body has to maintain a pH balance in order to function properly and prevent reflux and other digestive problems. In the digestive system, your saliva is in the 6.5 to 7.5 range, which makes it balanced. In the upper stomach, the acidity dips to 4.0 to start the breakdown of food, and then continues to become more acidic at 1.0 in the lower part of the stomach. The small intestine ranges from 4.0 to 7.0, which matches the colon.

Balancing Your Body's pH

In order to balance your body's pH, you need to get a reading of what your body's pH is before you make the decision of changing your body chemistry. You do this by purchasing a pH test and administering it when you urinate for the first time before you eat or drink anything. That is when you can get the most accurate reading. If your body registers in the highly acidic range, you need to look for foods that are alkaline in nature to bring it back into balance. Here is a short list of alkaline foods.

Alkaline foods

7.0-Neutral
- Butter
- Fresh cream with no salt
- Raw milk
- Most tap water (test yours to make sure)

8.0
- Apples
- Almonds
- Avocados
- Tomatoes
- Fresh corn
- Mushrooms
- Turnips
- Olives
- Soybeans
- Bell peppers
- Radishes
- Rhubarb
- Pineapple
- Cherries
- Millet
- Wild rice
- Strawberries
- Apricots
- Cantaloupe
- Honeydew

- Peaches
- Oranges
- Grapefruit
- Bananas

9.0
- Olive oil
- Herbal tea
- Sprouted grains
- Green tea
- Borage oil
- Raw zucchini
- Papayas
- Figs
- Blueberries
- Raw peas
- Most lettuce
- Raw eggplant
- Raw green beans
- Beets
- Greens
- Alfalfa sprouts
- Pears
- Mangoes
- Melons
- Kiwi
- Dates
- Sweet potato
- Tangerines

- Grapes

10.0
- Raw spinach
- Collards
- Artichokes
- Red cabbage
- Carrots
- Raw celery
- Cauliflower
- Raw broccoli
- Potato skins
- Asparagus
- Lemons
- Alfalfa grass
- Brussels sprouts
- Cucumbers
- Seaweed
- Onions
- Limes

Things to take note

On your road to bringing you body back into balance, there are a few things to keep in mind:

• To counteract 1 part of acidity in the body, you need to intake 20 parts of foods and liquids that are alkaline in nature.

• Some of the foods on the alkaline chart will become acidic when cooked.

• The best way to intake some of the foods on the chart is raw, such as in salads.

Chapter 3 - Adjusting Your Diet

I know I briefly covered this in the previous chapter, but it needs to expand a bit. There are foods which will trigger reflux, and we will discuss some of those here. I will also cover some foods that can help when an attack comes on.

Foods to avoid

High-acid foods

Most people think oranges and tomatoes, and they would be correct, but there are more foods that are acidic to consider. Any food that is high in citric acid or ascorbic acid (Vitamin C) can also trigger reflux. Some people will shy away from drinking orange juice because of the pain it induces, but most of the juice is concentrated. There are a couple of companies that do not make orange juice concentrated. The "Simply" brand is one. There are people I know that can drink the juices from that company, in small servings, and not have reflux.

Spicy foods

Everyone loves a good chili and others a good spicy curry or soup, but the enzymes and acidic nature of the spices can trigger reflux, leaving you in agony.

Onions and Garlic

These are two foods that can vary between people. Some can eat them with no problem, others in small doses, and others not at all. There is an enzyme in both can may cause flare-ups.

Caffeine

Coffee, soft drinks, chocolate all have one thing in common. They all contain caffeine. It could be the caffeine that can spark a flare-up, and in soft drinks, it could also be the carbonation.

Mint

This can be a trigger for some and not be one for others.

Foods that help

We all hate the list of foods we have to avoid, but did you know there were foods out there that help to curve, prevent, or in some cases, stop a flare-up? Here you go.

Oatmeal

Oatmeal is filling and can also help stave off a flare-up due to its ability to absorb liquids. It can also counter acid in foods like raisins and apples.

Ginger

Used in small bits, is can help with flare-ups as well as be a treatment for reflux. I know it seems counter-productive because of its acidic nature, but it is highly recommended for many digestive problems.

Aloe Vera

The juice from this plant can help with reflux other digestive problems.

Salads/salad greens

A good salad is alkaline in nature and can neutralize many acids in the stomach.

Banana

This is a fruit that is used to balance the pH in the system, reducing acidity.

Melon

This is another alkaline fruit that counters highly acidic foods.

Fennel

Usually used for seasoning, this herb is highly recommended for treating reflux. It also makes a good snack for those who like a licorice taste.

Chicken and Turkey

Boiled, baked, grilled, or sautéed without the skin.

Fish and seafood

Baked, grilled, sautéed, but not fried. Also wild caught would be preferable to farm raised.

Roots and Cruciferous Vegetables

Broccoli, green beans and the like are all great for those who suffer from reflex.

Parsley

Often the garnish on a plate in a high-end restaurant, chewing on a sprig of this can quell a reflux flare-up.

Papaya

This fruit contains an enzyme that can break down proteins into amino acids. It can also do wonders for acid reflux.

Water

Water is a very important substance. There is some advice on how to drink: food and water preferable take separately. In the morning it's good to take one cup of warm mineral water.

Chapter 4 - Herbal Supplements

In the natural health field, there are some herbs that you can either add to your food or take in capsule form to help with heartburn/reflux. You can even make some into a tea. We will go into that here.

Agrimony

You can use this herb to help with stomach upset and to help even out functions of the gastrointestinal tract. Agrimony is super effective in treating reflux, nausea, diarrhea, and vomiting.

Fenugreek seeds

This is a seed that creates a gel. This gel acts like a sponge, soaking up any excess acid in the system. The best part about these seeds is that they can be sprinkled on food and eaten with any preparation needed.

German Chamomile

This herb has been used for centuries to help with digestive issues including reflux and other heartburn issues. It is also good for general stomach pains.

Licorice

This herb not only helps with flare-ups, but it can also help heal damage done by reflux.

Slippery Elm

The bark of this tree has gelling properties that can absorb excess acid and other fluids, too. It can also sooth irritated stomach lining.

Turmeric

This herb has been found to have many healing properties, and they are finding more every day. Some discoveries include the ability to stop flare-ups, prevent future ones, arresting inflammation, and also instant relief of gas and bloating.

Recipes

Licorice and Chamomile Tea

1 tsp German Chamomile
1 tsp Licorice Root

- Bring two cups of water to a boil
- Add the licorice
- Reduce to medium boil for 15 minutes
- Place Chamomile in the pot
- Cover pot and steep for 10 minutes
- Strain out the herbs and add honey

Reflux Syrup

1/2 Ounce Slippery Elm
1/2 Ounce German Chamomile
1/2 Ounce Fenugreek Seeds
1/2 Ounce Fennel Root
1 Quart Water
2 Ounces Glycerin or Honey

- Add the herbs to the water.
- Boil the water down to a pint
- Strain out the herbs
- Add the honey or glycerin
- Mix well and let cool
- Take one tablespoon on flare-ups

Ginger Oil

8 Ounces Olive Oil
1 Ounce Ginger root

- Place in the Ginger and oil in a tinted glass bottle
- Close with a tight lid
- Leave in a cool dry place for two weeks
- Use in cooking recipes

Fennel and Fenugreek Oil

1 Ounces of Olive Oil
3 tbsp Fenugreek seeds
2 tbsp Dried Fennel
Follow instructions above

Digestion Oil

1/2 Ounce Agrimony
1/2 Ounce German Chamomile
1/2 Ounce Dried Fennel
1/2 Ounce Tumeric
1 Quart Water
2 Ounces Glycerin or Honey

- Add the herbs to the water.
- Boil the water down to a pint
- Strain out the herbs

- Add the honey or glycerin
- Mix well and let cool
- Take one tablespoon on flare-ups

Tips and Tricks

Baking Soda Trick

1 tsp Baking Soda
1/4 Cup water

- Dissolve the backing in the water
- Drink

There is a warning to this one. It does taste horrible. So have something to chase it with when you are done. You will burp, and as you burp, you will feel better. Depending on the severity, you may to do it more than once.

Peppermint

Though some would say mint makes it worse, peppermint can help a lot of many by cooling you from the inside out.

Sleep at an angle

Sleeping flat when you feel an attack coming is never a good idea. Sleep at a 45 degree angle for some relief until your treatment kicks in.

Exercise

This one is not as easy to do during a flare up, but walking will help get gasses moving and help you alleviate a flare-up along with any other treatments.

Food Diary

Log down all the foods you eat in a day, and log down your body's reactions to the food. If you have a flare up, make sure it's the actual type of you just ate and not one of the ingredients. Sometimes it's not the main part of the dish or side item, but a simple little ingredient that did it. Look for common ingredients.

Baking Soda

If you want to make pasta with marinara, but are dreading the burn after, put a pinch of baking soda in the sauce. The pinch should not be larger than half a pea size. Anymore and the sauce will taste funny. It will counteract the acid in the tomato sauce.

Herb Shops

In some herb shops or health foods stores, you will find papaya and mint tablets. These are normally chewable and work better than Tums and other antacids you can get at conventional stores. You can also find Fenugreek and fennel in capsules and by the ounce, too. These stores often sell pure Aloe Vera juice and all the herbs on the list in this chapter. Don't be afraid to ask the shop manager if there are other alternative as well.

Chapter 5 – Recipes to regulate the acidity

Here are some recipes you can try to regulate the acidity and help to regulate reflux.

Banana Nut Oatmeal

1/2 Cup Steel Cut Oats
1 1/2 Cups water
2 Medium Size Ripe bananas
1 tsp vanilla extract
1/2 tsp nutmeg
1/2 tsp cinnamon
1/8 Cup brown sugar
Pinch of salt

- Mash the bananas
- Mix the sugar, nutmeg, vanilla, and cinnamon into the bananas
- Bring the water to a boil
- Add the salt
- Stir in the banana mixture
- Let simmer for five minutes
- Bring it back to a boil and add the oats
- Simmer covered until soft, about 15 minutes

Grilled Chicken Salad

3 ounces grilled chicken, chopped
1/4 Cup raw Spinach
1/4 Cup Romaine Lettuce
1/4 cup Cucumber, peeled and chopped
1/4 Cup Baby Bella mushrooms, chopped
1/4 Cup sliced Strawberries
2 tbsp sliced Almonds
1 tbsp Olive Oil
1/2 lemon Juiced

- Mix the vegetables in a bowl
- Top with the chicken
- Drizzle the oil and lemon
- Toss once more and eat

Morning Juice

1/4 cup Zucchini
5 Strawberries
1/2 Pear
3 Sprigs of Parsley
1/2 Red Apple

Run all through a juicer and drink before your meal. It will help with digestion.

Yogurt Smoothie

1/2 cup yogurt
1 medium banana
1/4 papaya chunks
6 Strawberries
1/4 Cup Pineapple

Blend all in a blender and add ice to thicken.

Melon Salad

1/4 Cup Honeydew
1/4 Cup Cantaloupe
1/2 Cup Vanilla Yogurt

Mix together and eat as a snack or with a meal.

Even though the list of foods may seem limited, but there a lot of things you can do with the foods take keep your digestive system functioning normally. Challenge yourself by adding a food you've never tried before to your daily intake. Step out of your comfort zone. You will be surprised at the foods will like that you didn't think you would.

Chapter 6 – Stress

You can't fully address digestive problems without touching on one of the reasons our bodies are more prone to illness and disorders.

In our everyday lives, we encounter stress and stressful situations. Between paying bills, balancing budgets, balancing work with recreation, we tend to get overwhelmed. This causes stress. Here are some things you can do to reduce it.

Exercise

This can be anything from just taking a walk to joining a gym. Find a type of exercise you like, and you will be more likely to stick with it. Two highly recommended exercises are Yoga and Thai Chi.

Meditation

Mediating can be a great way to relieve stress. There are many ways to meditate, but if you would like an easy method, here is a quick guide to Fixed-Point Meditation:

• Light a candle or pick a spot on a wall to concentrate on.

• Breathe in slowly as you isolate and tighten a muscle group.

• Exhale slowly as you relax the muscle group, concentrating on the point you chose to focus on.

• Repeat the process until you have tightened and relaxed all of the muscles in your body.

Read a Book

Sometimes the best way to relieve stress is to immerse yourself in something that sparks your imagination. Reading a book does just that. A good book will keep your attention focused on the story and provide you the break you need from the everyday stresses.

Spoil Yourself

We tend to get so wrapped up in caring for others we forget to pamper ourselves. A soak in a tub, a trip to a spa for a massage or facial treatment can be great ways to pamper and spoil you.

Take Up a Hobby

Find something you like doing, like drawing, writing, or even crafting. Taking up a hobby can also take your mind of stress.

Unplug

This may be the hardest one on the list to do, but you are exposing your mind to constant stimulus when you check your social media, emails, surf the web and even text. Designate a time during the day to unplug all electronics and just do something that does not need a computer to do. A few suggestions have been listed above.

Play/Hang Out

Take time out of your day to play with your kids if you have a family or make dates to hang out with friends to talk or have fun. Either one will help you relieve stress and help you be healthy.

In this book you can find some advice how to improve your situation, but don't forget if you want to solve your problem you must find a reason. **So it's better to start from a medical examination.**

Medical advice

If you suffer from acid reflux it can be a signal that you have some problems in your body.

1. *Check your liver and pancreas and stomach.*

   The process of food digestion is very complicated. There are lots of substances (such as enzymes, HCl) used in digestion process and there is a balance between them). When the balance is broken you can get some negative consequences such as reflux. So it's recommended to visit your physician. He can advise you to make Esophagogastroduodenoscopy or get some tests.

2. *Check if you have food intolerance*

   Get IgG4 testing food intolerance?

3. *Check if you have Helicobacter Pylori*

   Get a blood test IgG on Helicobacter Pylori.

4. *Try to avoid non-steroidal anti-inflammatory drugs or antibiotics.*

Conclusion

Your digestive system is a fine balance and keeping it sometimes can be hard to do, but I hope some of the advice in this book can help you gain a healthier digestive system and live a fuller life. Until next time, be happy and be healthy.